Reverse Type 1 Diabetes

A Comprehensive Guide to Reversing and Managing Type 1 Diabetes Naturally

Table Of Contents:

<u>Introduction:</u>

Type 1 diabetes is a resolved condition that influences a massive number of individuals from one side of the world to the other.

It is portrayed by the obliteration of insulin-conveying cells in the pancreas, inciting a weakness to make sufficient insulin to facilitate glucose levels.

The recognizable strategy for overseeing directing sort 1 diabetes consolidates a mix of insulin implantations, seeing of blood glucose levels, and adherence to an outrageous eating routine and work-out day to day plan.

Regardless, different people are usually looking for elective ways to deal with their condition.

In this all out partner, we will investigate trading type 1 diabetes and give a manual for those hoping to contemplate their condition in a more sweeping and customary manner.

We will cover different bits of type 1 diabetes, including its causes, delayed consequences, and standard treatment choices, as well as bounce into top tier examination and elective approaches to dealing with this condition.

Through a mix of master experiences, reasonable tips, and invigorating individual stories, we desire to enable those with type 1 diabetes to anticipate command over their success and go on with a full and satisfying life.

Whether you are not permanently set up or have been living to have type 1 diabetes for a surprisingly long time, this guide offers one more point of view and a flood of data that can help you on your excursion to better success.

Thus, in the event that you are prepared to even more significantly focus on trading and overseeing type 1 diabetes consistently, we should start.

Chapter 1: Introduction To Type 1 Diabetes

Type 1 diabetes, generally called juvenile diabetes or insulin-subordinate diabetes, is a persevering condition that impacts how your body processes glucose (glucose).

Glucose is a critical wellspring of energy for your body, yet it needs insulin to enter your telephones.

In type 1 diabetes, your protected structure mistakenly attacks and wrecks the telephones in your pancreas that produce insulin, called beta cells.

This prompts a lack of insulin in your body, causing your glucose levels to rise unreasonably high.

The particular justification behind type 1 diabetes is dark, yet being a mix of innate and normal variables is acknowledged.

It normally occurs in children, adolescents, or energetic adults, and requires well established treatment with insulin mixtures or the usage of an insulin siphon.

The symptoms of type 1 diabetes can outgrow no place and include:

1. Extended thirst and craving
2. Standard pee
3. Ridiculous exhaustion
4. Clouded vision
5. Astounding weight decrease

If left untreated, high glucose levels can incite serious ailments, for instance, coronary sickness, nerve hurt, visual inadequacy, kidney disillusionment, and evacuations.

Anyway, with authentic organization, people with type 1 diabetes can have sound and dynamic presences.

This incorporates checking glucose levels reliably, following a strong eating normal, working out, and tolerating insulin as supported by a clinical benefits provider.

Chapter 2: Definition And Causes Of Type 1 Diabetes

Type 1 diabetes, otherwise called adolescent diabetes or insulin-subordinate diabetes, is a persistent immune system sickness portrayed by the obliteration of the beta cells in the pancreas liable for delivering insulin.

Subsequently, individuals with type 1 diabetes can't deliver insulin and have to depend on customary infusions of insulin or an insulin siphon to control their glucose levels.

The specific reason for type 1 diabetes is obscure, however being a blend of hereditary and ecological factors is accepted.

Some examination recommends that a viral contamination or openness to specific ecological poisons might set off the resistant framework to assault and obliterate the beta cells in the pancreas.

Different investigations recommend a hereditary inclination to fostering the sickness, which might be set off by ecological factors like a viral contamination or openness to specific poisons.

No matter what the particular reason, the outcome is something very similar: an individual with type 1 diabetes can't deliver insulin, which prompts raised glucose levels and an expanded gamble of different medical conditions, including coronary illness, stroke, nerve harm, kidney harm, and eye issues.

People with type 1 diabetes genuinely should screen their glucose levels consistently and to keep a solid eating routine and way of life, including customary active work and insulin treatment, to assist with dealing with the infection and diminish their gamble of inconveniences.

Chapter 3: Symptoms And Diagnosis Of Type 1 Diabetes

Type 1 diabetes is an immune system sickness where the body's safe framework assaults and obliterates the insulin-creating cells in the pancreas, known as beta cells.

This prompts a lack of insulin, which is expected to direct glucose levels.

Normal side effects of type 1 diabetes include:

1. Expanded thirst
2. Incessant pee
3. Outrageous craving
4. Weight reduction
5. Weariness
6. Peevishness
7. Obscured vision
8. Slow-mending cuts and injuries
9. Shivering or deadness in the hands and feet
10. Incessant contaminations

Finding of type 1 diabetes is normally made in view of side effects and the consequences of blood tests that action glucose levels.

A fasting plasma glucose (FPG) test, an oral glucose resilience test (OGTT), or a hemoglobin A1C test can be utilized to analyze diabetes.

At times, a specialist may likewise play out an irregular plasma glucose test. On the off chance that the consequences of these tests are high, a specialist might play out extra tests to affirm the determination of type 1 diabetes.

It's critical to take note of the fact that certain individuals with type 1 diabetes might not have any side effects whatsoever, or may have gentle side effects that slip through the cracks.

That is the reason it's critical to have normal check-ups with your medical care supplier to screen your glucose levels and guarantee that your diabetes is all around controlled.

Chapter 4: Importance Of Reversing Type 1 Diabetes

Reversing Type 1 diabetes is important for several reasons:

- Improved health: Reversing Type 1 diabetes can help improve overall health and prevent the onset of complications associated with the disease, such as heart disease, kidney failure, nerve damage, and eye problems.

- Enhanced quality of life: Reversing Type 1 diabetes can help individuals manage their blood sugar levels more effectively, reducing the need for frequent injections of insulin pump therapy, and leading to improved energy levels, better sleep, and reduced stress.

- Cost savings: Reversing Type 1 diabetes can lead to cost savings over the long term, as individuals are less likely to require medical interventions, hospitalizations, and other treatments associated with complications.

- Better mental health: Reversing Type 1 diabetes can help improve mental health, reducing the stress and anxiety associated with managing the disease on a daily basis.

- Increased independence: Reversing Type 1 diabetes can help individuals gain more control over their health, allowing them to live a more independent life without being constantly dependent on medication and medical interventions.

It's important to note that reversing Type 1 diabetes is not currently possible with existing treatments.

However, researchers are actively working to develop new treatments that may one day be able to reverse the disease.

In the meantime, individuals with Type 1 diabetes can work with their healthcare team to manage the disease and prevent complications through careful blood sugar control and a healthy lifestyle.

Chapter 5: Understanding The Body's Response To Type 1 Diabetes

Type 1 diabetes is an ongoing immune system infection that influences the manner in which the body delivers and uses insulin, a chemical that manages glucose levels.

In Type 1 diabetes, the resistant framework erroneously assaults and annihilates the insulin-delivering cells in the pancreas, called beta cells.

This prompts a total absence of insulin in the body, and the requirement for everyday infusions or utilization of an insulin siphon to deal with the condition.

At the point when there is an absence of insulin, the body can't really move glucose (sugar) from the circulation system into the cells, where it is utilized for energy.

Thus, glucose levels in the blood rise, prompting high glucose (hyperglycemia).

This can prompt side effects like expanded thirst, continuous pee, weakness, and obscured vision.

To make up for the absence of insulin, the body begins to separate fats and muscle tissue for energy, which can prompt weight reduction and muscle squandering.

The elevated degrees of glucose in the blood can likewise make arm veins and organs over the long haul, prompting long haul confusions, for example, coronary illness, nerve harm, and eye issues.

People with Type 1 diabetes really should intently screen their glucose levels and change their insulin dosages as needs be.

Eating a decent eating routine, remaining genuinely dynamic, and overseeing feelings of anxiety can likewise assist with dealing with the condition and forestall intricacies.

Ordinary check-ups with a medical services supplier are likewise critical to screen for any possible inconveniences and to guarantee powerful administration of the condition.

Chapter 6: The Role Of Insulin In Reversing Type 1 Diabetes

Insulin assumes an essential part in switching Type 1 Diabetes.

Type 1 Diabetes is an immune system sickness where the body's safe framework obliterates the insulin-delivering cells (beta cells) in the pancreas, prompting a lack of insulin.

This prompts a development of glucose in the circulatory system, which can cause serious medical issues over the long haul.

To oversee Type 1 Diabetes, individuals with this condition should accept insulin infusions or utilize an insulin siphon to give the vital insulin their bodies need to control glucose levels.

The objective of insulin treatment is to keep up with as near ordinary glucose levels as could really be expected, which assists with decreasing the gamble of growing long haul complexities related with high glucose levels, for example, coronary illness, nerve harm, visual deficiency, and kidney infection.

While insulin infusions or siphon treatment can assist with overseeing Type 1 Diabetes, it doesn't invert the condition.

Presently, there is no solution for Type 1 Diabetes, and individuals with the condition should accept insulin until the end of their lives.

Notwithstanding, with legitimate administration and control of glucose levels, individuals with Type 1 Diabetes can have solid and dynamic existences.

Chapter 7: The Impact Of Type 1 diabetes On The Body

Type 1 diabetes is a constant ailment that influences the body's capacity to deliver insulin, a chemical that controls glucose levels.

The body's resistant framework assaults and obliterates the cells in the pancreas liable for delivering insulin, prompting a total absence of insulin creation.

Without insulin, glucose (sugar) gathers in the circulatory system, prompting high glucose levels (hyperglycemia).

This can adversely affect the body, including:

- Harmed veins and nerves: Over the long run, high glucose levels can harm the veins and nerves in the eyes, kidneys, heart, and different organs, prompting serious medical issues like visual deficiency, kidney illness, coronary illness, and neuropathy (nerve harm).

- Expanded chance of contaminations: High glucose levels can debilitate the insusceptible framework, making it more challenging for the body to battle diseases.

- Lack of hydration: Unnecessary pee because of high glucose levels can prompt parchedness, which can cause weariness, unsteadiness, and different side effects.

- Ketoacidosis: In extreme cases, the absence of insulin can prompt a perilous condition called diabetic ketoacidosis (DKA), where the body starts to separate fat for energy rather than glucose, delivering overabundance ketones that can develop in the circulation system and lead to a risky corrosive base irregularity.

To deal with the effects of type 1 diabetes, people really should screen their glucose levels, accept insulin as recommended, eat a sound eating routine, participate in normal active work, and work with their medical care group to deal with the condition.

Chapter 8: Understanding The Immune System And Autoimmunity

Type 1 diabetes is a constant ailment that influences the body's capacity to deliver insulin, a chemical that controls glucose levels.

The body's resistant framework assaults and obliterates the cells in the pancreas liable for delivering insulin, prompting a total absence of insulin creation.

Without insulin, glucose (sugar) gathers in the circulatory system, prompting high glucose levels (hyperglycemia).

This can adversely affect the body, including:

- Harmed veins and nerves: Over the long run, high glucose levels can harm the veins and nerves in the eyes, kidneys, heart, and different organs, prompting serious medical issues like visual deficiency, kidney illness, coronary illness, and neuropathy (nerve harm).

- Expanded chance of contaminations: High glucose levels can debilitate the insusceptible framework, making it more challenging for the body to battle diseases.

- Lack of hydration: Unnecessary pee because of high glucose levels can prompt parchedness, which can cause weariness, unsteadiness, and different side effects.

- Ketoacidosis: In extreme cases, the absence of insulin can prompt a perilous condition called diabetic ketoacidosis (DKA), where the body starts to separate fat for energy rather than glucose, delivering overabundance ketones that can develop in the circulation system and lead to a risky corrosive base irregularity.

To deal with the effects of type 1 diabetes, people really should screen their glucose levels, accept insulin as recommended, eat a sound eating routine, participate in normal active work, and work with their medical care group to deal with the condition.

<u>Chapter 9: Lifestyle Changes For Reversing Type 1 Diabetes</u>

Pivoting type 1 diabetes is crazy, as a resistant framework ailment wrecks the insulin-conveying cells in the pancreas.

Regardless, there are a couple of lifestyle changes that can help people with type 1 diabetes manage their condition and work on their overall prosperity:

- Shrewd slimming down: Eating a fair and nutritious eating routine, including a great deal of natural items, vegetables, whole grains, and lean protein, can help with overseeing glucose levels and work on by and large prosperity.

- Genuine work: Typical real work, similar to action or vivacious walking, can help with cutting down glucose levels and further foster insulin responsiveness.

- Checking glucose levels: Standard seeing of glucose levels is a critical piece of managing type 1 diabetes.

This ought to be conceivable using a glucometer, which gauges how much glucose in the blood.

- Medication the board: Taking insulin implantations or using an insulin guide as composed by an expert can help with coordinating glucose levels and hinder troubles.

- Stress the board: Stress can impact glucose levels and make it hard to direct kind 1 diabetes. Stress-the leaders strategies, as significant breathing, thought, and yoga, can help with chipping away at by and large prosperity and regulate sensations of uneasiness.

- Incredible rest inclinations: Getting adequate quality rest is critical for supervising type 1 diabetes.

  Hold back nothing of significant length of rest each night and lay out a rest supportive environment.

- Standard check-ups: Typical check-ups with a clinical consideration provider can assist screen for any snares and make changes as per treatment relying upon the circumstance.

It's indispensable to observe that everyone with type 1 diabetes is remarkable, and what works for one individual may not work for another.

It's basic to work personally with a clinical consideration provider to encourage an organization plan that is great for you.

<u>Chapter 10: Diet And Nutrition For Reversing Type 1 Diabetes</u>

Diet and nourishment assume an essential part in keeping up with generally wellbeing and health.

An even eating regimen ought to incorporate different supplement thick food varieties, including organic products, vegetables, entire grains, lean proteins, and sound fats.

A few vital supplements to zero in on include:

- Carbs: the body's essential wellspring of energy, found in food varieties like organic products, vegetables, grains, and dairy items.

- Proteins: significant for building and fixing tissues, found in food sources like meat, poultry, fish, beans, and dairy items.

- Fats: essential for cerebrum capability and keeping up with sound cell films, found in food varieties like avocados, nuts, seeds, and olive oil.

- Nutrients and Minerals: significant for different physical processes, found in many food varieties including natural products, vegetables, dairy items, and entire grains.

It is likewise vital to restrict your admission of added sugars, immersed and trans fats, and sodium.

Drinking a lot of water and remaining genuinely dynamic are likewise fundamental parts of a solid eating regimen and way of life.

It's critical to take note of that everybody's wholesome necessities are one of a kind and can be impacted by elements like age, orientation, weight, and actual work levels.

Counseling an enrolled dietitian or specialist can assist you with deciding the best dietary methodology for you.

Chapter 11: Exercise And Physical Activity For Reversing Type 1 Diabetes

Practice and active work can be advantageous for individuals with type 1 diabetes.

Standard active work can assist with further developing insulin responsiveness and glucose control, which can assist with decreasing the gamble of long haul entanglements.

Be that as it may, it's critical to screen blood glucose levels previously, during, and after actual work, as practicing can influence glucose levels in various ways, contingent upon variables, for example, the sort and power of the action, insulin portions, and diet.

Here are a few hints for individuals with type 1 diabetes who need to work out:

- Work with your PCP or diabetes group to make an arrangement that turns out best for you.

  This can assist with guaranteeing your security and viable glucose control while working out.

- Check your blood glucose levels previously, during, and after active work.

- On the off chance that your blood glucose levels are low, have a fast wellspring of sugars (like natural product juice, candy, or a glucose gel) close by to raise your levels.

- In the event that your levels are high, hold on until they descend prior to beginning actual work.

- Wear clinical ID (ID) in the event of a crisis.

- Hydrate previously, during, and after actual work to forestall drying out.

- Make a point to change insulin dosages in view of the sort and force of the movement and your glucose levels.

Keep in mind, active work ought to be a standard piece of your general diabetes board plan, however it's vital to screen glucose levels and work with your primary care physician to foster that employer.

Chapter 12: Stress Management And Sleep For Reversing Type 1 Diabetes

Overseeing pressure and getting sufficient rest can assist people with the condition better deal with their side effects and work on their general wellbeing.

Stress can influence glucose levels and disturb the body's chemical equilibrium, making it harder to oversee diabetes.

To assist with overseeing pressure, it is critical to take part in unwinding procedures, like profound breathing, contemplation, and exercise.

Normal actual work can likewise assist with lessening pressure and work on in general wellbeing.

Sufficient rest is likewise significant for people with type 1 diabetes, as it directs chemicals and further develops glucose control.

Absence of rest can cause changes in chemicals and glucose levels, which can make it challenging to oversee diabetes.

It is prescribed to hold back nothing long stretches of rest each evening and lay out a reliable rest plan.

While stress the board and rest can't switch type 1 diabetes, they can assist individuals with better dealing with their side effects and work on their general wellbeing.

People with type 1 diabetes should work with their medical services group to foster a far reaching board plan that incorporates way of life changes and clinical therapy to deal with their condition.

Chapter 13: Quitting Smoking And Reducing Alcohol Consumption For Reversing Type 1 Diabetes

As a sort 1 diabetic patient, stopping smoking and lessening liquor utilization is significant in light of multiple factors:

- Hazard of Complexities: Smoking and over the top liquor utilization increment the gamble of creating intricacies like cardiovascular illness, fringe neuropathy, and diabetic retinopathy.

- Glucose Control: Smoking and liquor utilization can adversely affect glucose control, which is particularly significant for individuals with diabetes.

  Liquor can cause vacillations in glucose levels, while smoking can influence insulin responsiveness.

- Mending: Smoking and unnecessary liquor utilization can defer recuperating and increment the gamble of contaminations, which can be especially risky for individuals with diabetes who may as of now have a compromised safe framework.

- Way of life The board: Keeping a solid way of life is significant for overseeing diabetes. Stopping smoking and diminishing liquor utilization can work on by and large wellbeing and prosperity, making it more straightforward to deal with the infection.

- Better Wellbeing: Stopping smoking and decreasing liquor utilization has various medical advantages, including working on cardiovascular wellbeing, diminished hazard of malignant growth, and worked on liver capability.

In this way, stopping smoking and lessening liquor utilization can enormously help the wellbeing and the board of type 1 diabetes.

Assuming you're experiencing issues stopping, there are numerous assets accessible to help, including support gatherings, nicotine substitution treatment, and advising.

Chapter 14: Alternative Therapies For Reversing Type 1 Diabetes

There are a couple of elective medicines that have been proposed to help with regulating secondary effects and conceivably further foster outcomes.

In any case, it's basic to observe that countless of these medicines have confined consistent verification to help their practicality, and some could attempt to be disastrous.

The following are a couple of elective medicines that have been proposed for type 1 diabetes:

- Diet: Certain people with type 1 diabetes follow uncommon eating regimens, for instance, the high-fat, low-carb ketogenic diet, with the assumption that it will additionally foster their glucose control.

  In any case, there is confined consistent confirmation to help this system, and serious dietary changes can be attempting to stay aware of long term.

- Local fixes: Certain people with type 1 diabetes use regular fixes, similar to cinnamon or upsetting melon, to help with managing their secondary effects.

  Nevertheless, there is confined coherent evidence to help the usage of these fixes, and some could communicate with prescriptions or have other ominous effects.

- Needle treatment: Certain people with type 1 diabetes have endeavored needle treatment with the assumption that it will additionally foster their glucose control.

  Nevertheless, there is limited legitimate verification to help the usage of needle treatment thus, and more investigation is supposed to choose its feasibility.

- Chiropractic: Certain people with type 1 diabetes have endeavored chiropractic medications with the assumption that they will additionally foster their glucose control.

  In any case, there is confined consistent confirmation to help the use of chiropractic thus, and more assessment is supposed to choose its feasibility.

It makes a big difference to speak with your clinical consideration provider before endeavoring any elective medicines for type 1 diabetes.

They can help you with checking the normal benefits and risks of these systems and assurance that any treatment you get is safeguarded and strong.

Chapter 15: Clinical Interventions For Reversing Type 1 Diabetes

Islet cell Transplant For Reversing Type 1 Diabetes:

Islet cell transplantation is a promising treatment for type 1 diabetes, a condition wherein the body's protected design assaults and wrecks the insulin-secretion beta cells in the pancreas.

In islet cell transplantation, bound islets (heaps of cells) are taken from a supplier pancreas and moved into the liver of the individual with diabetes.

Right when the moved islets are working, they produce insulin and transport it considering glucose levels in the blood.

This course glucose levels, diminishing the fundamentals for standard insulin blends and working on individual satisfaction for individuals with type 1 diabetes.

After a short time, islet cell transplantation is currently viewed as exploratory and isn't exactly accessible.

It is in general utilized for individuals with type 1 diabetes who have serious hypoglycemia (low glucose) or who have not had the decision to accomplish stunning glucose control with insulin treatment.

The point of view is tangled and requires a party of specialists in transplantation and diabetes care.

Moreover, islet cell transplantation moderately requires a lifetime obligation to ingesting immunosuppressive answers for forestall dismissal of the moved cells, which can make serious unconstrained impacts.

This treatment is right at this point being dissected and its long adequacy and security are not yet completely figured out.

With everything considered, while islet cell transplantation shows guarantee as a treatment for type 1 diabetes, it is right, eventually tried to be exploratory and isn't normally open.

Individuals with type 1 diabetes ought to visit with their clinical thought supplier about the sensible advantages and dangers of islet cell transplantation and whether it might be a fair choice for them.

Stem cell Therapy For Reversing Type 1 Diabetes:

Undifferentiated cell treatment has been proposed as an expected treatment for Type 1 diabetes.

This is on the grounds that immature microorganisms can separate into various kinds of cells, including insulin-delivering beta cells.

In principle, bringing new undifferentiated cells into the body of an individual with Type 1 diabetes could assist with reestablishing the individual's capacity to create insulin and manage their glucose levels.

Nonetheless, foundational microorganism treatment for Type 1 diabetes is as yet viewed as trial and isn't yet broadly accessible.

There have been a few clinical preliminaries examining the utilization of undifferentiated organisms for treating Type 1 diabetes, however the outcomes have been blended and more examination is expected to decide the security and viability of this methodology.

It is likewise vital to take note that foundational microorganism treatment for Type 1 diabetes isn't a fix and won't invert the hidden immune system process that prompts the obliteration of the individual's own insulin-creating beta cells.

Subsequently, individuals with Type 1 diabetes will in any case have to deal with their condition through insulin treatment, diet, and way of life adjustments regardless of whether they get foundational microorganism treatment.

Chapter 16: Experimental Therapies And Clinical Trials For Reversing Type 1 Diabetes

There are a couple of exploratory medicines and clinical starters underway to inverse or fix Type 1 diabetes conceivably. Indisputably the most uplifting philosophies include:

- Islet cell transplantation: This treatment incorporates moving insulin-making cells called islets into the body.

  Though this approach has shown safety in little primers, it stays preliminary and requires mindful organization to hinder excusal of the moved cells.

- Central microorganism treatment: This approach means to recuperate hurt or destroyed insulin-making cells by using undifferentiated creatures.

  Researchers are examining various wellsprings of undifferentiated organic entities, recollecting those found for the pancreas, as well as actuated pluripotent juvenile microorganisms produced using the patient's own telephones.

- Lymphocyte treatment: This approach incorporates changing the patient's safe system to hold it back from pursuing the body's own insulin-making cells.

  One promising technique is to plan Safe framework microorganisms to see and destroy unequivocal cells that cause resistant framework demolition of islets.

- Beta cell recuperation: This approach means to enliven the turn of events and capacity of new insulin-making cells in the pancreas.

  Experts are examining various procedures to achieve this, including the usage of improvement factors, little iotas, and inherited controls.

- Immune opposition acknowledgment: This approach plans to "train" the resistant structure to stop pursuing insulin-conveying cells.

  Experts are researching various frameworks for achieving this, including the usage of quieting drugs and immunomodulatory trained professionals.

It implies a considerable amount to observe that these procedures are still to start with periods of progress and more assessment is expected before they can be comprehensively embraced as medications for Type 1 diabetes.
Incidentally, they expect a fix or reversal of this steady condition from here onward.

Chapter 17: Insulin Pump Therapy And Continuous Glucose Monitoring For Reversing Type 1 Diabetes

Insulin siphon treatment and persevering glucose noticing (CGM) are two normally elaborate methodologies for directing Kind 1 diabetes.

Type 1 diabetes is a continuous condition where the pancreas can't make insulin, a substance that coordinates glucose levels.

Insulin siphon treatment gives a strategy for conveying insulin in a more physiological and versatile manner, when diverged from different regular mixtures.

The insulin siphon is a little device that is worn outside the body and can be altered to convey insulin considering changes in glucose levels.

Persevering glucose noticing (CGM) is a device that reliably checks glucose levels in the interstitial fluid under the skin.

CGMs give steady information about glucose levels and help with perceiving examples, models, and high or low glucose levels.

This information can be used to make acclimations to insulin segments and to help with hindering outrageous hypoglycemia or hyperglycemia.

Both insulin siphon treatment and CGM can additionally foster glucose control and individual fulfillment for people with Type 1 diabetes.

Regardless, it's crucial to observe that these developments are not an answer for the condition and require advancing self-organization, including standard noticing and changes as per insulin segments.

Likewise, both insulin siphon treatment and CGM have anticipated risks and weaknesses, so it is basic to check the benefits and risks while picking the choice about whether to use them.

These developments really should not be fitting for everyone with Type 1 diabetes, and a clinical benefits provider should be guided to choose the best technique for individual necessities.

Chapter 18: Managing Type 1 Diabetes

Type 1 diabetes is an ongoing condition that requires cautious administration to hold glucose levels under tight restraints.

Here are a few general ways to oversee Type 1 diabetes:

- Observing glucose levels: Checking your glucose levels consistently with a glucose meter is a significant piece of overseeing Type 1 diabetes.

- Taking insulin infusions: Individuals with Type 1 diabetes need to take insulin infusions a few times each day or utilize an insulin siphon to keep up with typical glucose levels.

- Eating a fair eating regimen: It's critical to eat a decent eating routine that incorporates a blend of starches, protein, and solid fats.

  It's likewise useful to eat ordinary, little dinners over the course of the day to assist with keeping up with stable glucose levels.

- Remaining dynamic: Ordinary actual work can assist with controlling glucose levels and diminish the gamble of long haul inconveniences related with Type 1 diabetes.

- Overseeing pressure: Stress can influence glucose levels, so it means a lot to track down solid ways of overseeing pressure, like through exercise, contemplation, or conversing with a specialist.

- Checking for confusions: Individuals with Type 1 diabetes are in danger of creating complexities, like diabetic retinopathy, neuropathy, and nephropathy.

  Standard check-ups with a specialist can help distinguish and deal with these entanglements.

- Remaining coordinated: Monitoring your glucose levels, insulin portions, and other significant data can assist you with keeping steady over your diabetes.

  Consider utilizing a logbook or a portable application to monitor your data.

It's vital to work intimately with a medical care supplier to foster a diabetes plan that turns out best for you.

Chapter 19: Monitoring Blood Sugar Levels When Reversing Type 1 Diabetes

Observing glucose levels is a significant part of overseeing Type 1 diabetes, as it assists people with understanding how their body is answering insulin and different meds, as well as concerning the food they eat.

By consistently estimating their glucose levels, individuals with Type 1 diabetes can change their insulin portions, food decisions, and actual work to keep their glucose inside an objective reach and keep away from long haul complexities.

There are multiple ways of observing glucose levels, including:

- Fingerstick testing: This is the most widely recognized method for observing glucose levels, and includes utilizing a little gadget called a glucometer to get a drop of blood from the fingertip.

  The blood is then put on a test strip and embedded into the glucometer, which gives a perusal of the ongoing glucose level.

- Nonstop glucose observing (CGM): This includes wearing a little sensor under the skin that actions glucose levels in the liquid between cells.
The sensor sends readings to a showcase gadget, taking into consideration constant checking of glucose levels.

- A1C test: This test estimates the typical glucose level over a few months. It is finished in a research center and doesn't need fasting or halting insulin.

It's essential to take note of that observing glucose levels is only one part of overseeing Type 1 diabetes, and it ought to be finished related to different measures like a fair eating regimen, normal active work, and accepting insulin as recommended by a medical care supplier.

Chapter 20: Managing Hypoglycemia And Hyperglycemia When Reversing Type 1 Diabetes

Hypoglycemia and hyperglycemia are the two circumstances connected with glucose levels.

Hypoglycemia is a condition where the glucose levels fall underneath ordinary, while hyperglycemia is a condition where the glucose levels are raised better than average.

Overseeing hypoglycemia:

1. Eat little, regular feasts and snacks over the course of the day to keep glucose levels stable.
2. Abstain from skipping dinners or standing by excessively lengthy feasts.
3. Incorporate a wellspring of protein with every feast and nibble to slow the processing of sugars.
4. Pick complex starches, like entire grains, natural products, and vegetables, rather than basic carbs, like treats, pop, and other sweet food varieties.

5. Screen glucose levels consistently and convey a wellspring of glucose, like natural product juice or hard sweets, to treat low glucose levels in the event that they happen.

Overseeing hyperglycemia:

1. Follow a fair and reliable feast plan with set times for eating and set bits of food.
2. Pick better carb choices, like organic products, vegetables, and entire grains, and cut off sweet and handled food sources.
3. Screen glucose levels consistently and change meds as coordinated by a specialist.
4. Take part in standard actual work, as suggested by a specialist.
5. Abstain from skipping dinners or defers in eating.

It means a lot to work with a medical care supplier to foster an individualized administration plan for hypoglycemia or hyperglycemia, as every individual's requirements might change.

<u>Chapter 21: Adapting To A Low-Carbohydrate Diet When Reversing Type 1 Diabetes</u>

Type 1 diabetes is a steady condition that impacts how your body processes sugar (glucose).

While there is no known answer for type 1 diabetes, certain people with the condition have had accomplishment managing their glucose levels by following a low-carb diet.

A low-carb diet incorporates diminishing how much sugars you eat, as carbs separate into glucose in the body.

By eating less carbs, you can help with overseeing how much glucose in your course framework and cut off the prerequisite for insulin implantations.

The following are a couple of ways of acclimating to a low-carb diet for type 1 diabetes:

- Counsel a subject matter expert or enrolled dietitian: Before carrying out any enhancements to your eating schedule, it's basic to chat with your essential consideration doctor or an enlisted dietitian.

They can help you with choosing the ideal extent of carbs for your particular necessities.

- Plan your meals: Dining experience organizing is a critical piece of a low-carb diet. Plan and guarantee you have the right food assortments accessible to make low-carb feasts.

  Avoid dealing with food sources and actually pick new vegetables, proteins, and strong fats.

- Screen your glucose levels: Reliably checking your glucose levels is essential for managing type 1 diabetes.

  Your PCP or dietitian can help you with choosing the right repeat of testing and what to look for in your results.

- Stay hydrated: Drinking a ton of water is critical on a low-carb diet, as the body would convey more water as it polishes off fat.

- Be prepared for the "low-carb flu": When you first begin a low-carb diet, you could experience a couple of incidental effects like headache, fatigue, and dourness.

These aftereffects are regularly insinuated as the "low-carb flu" and are fleeting.

It's vital to observe that a low-carb diet is surely not a one-size-fits-all response for type 1 diabetes.
It makes a big difference to work with your essential doctor or enlisted dietitian to encourage that business and help you with managing your glucose levels, as a matter of fact.

Chapter 22: Making Lifestyle Changes And Staying Motivated When Reversing Type 1 Diabetes

Making way of life changes and remaining inspired are critical for overseeing and switching type 1 diabetes. Here are a few hints that might be useful:

- Foster a good dieting plan: A solid eating regimen is a significant piece of overseeing type 1 diabetes.

  Counsel an enrolled dietitian for a dinner plan that is custom fitted to your particular necessities and objectives.

- Work-out consistently: Normal active work can assist with controlling glucose levels and further develop insulin responsiveness.

  Find an activity that you appreciate, like swimming, climbing, or yoga, and go for the gold of moderate movement most days of the week.

- Oversee pressure: Stress can cause changes in glucose levels, so it means quite a bit to track down solid ways of overseeing pressure.

  This might incorporate rehearsing unwinding methods, like profound breathing or contemplation.

- Get sufficient rest: Go for long periods of rest every evening.

  Absence of rest can influence glucose levels and increment the gamble of creating other medical conditions.

- Keep tabs on your development: Keep a log of your glucose levels, food consumption, and actual work.

  This can assist you with recognizing examples and make vital acclimations to your way of life.

- Interface with others: Associate with other people who have type 1 diabetes. Joining a care group or online local area can give a feeling of local area, backing, and support.

- Track down an inspiration: Find something that causes you to adhere to your way of life changes, for example, a longing to work on your wellbeing, feel significantly improved, or stay away from intricacies from diabetes.

Keep in mind, putting forth a way of life changes takes time and effort, yet the advantages are worth the effort.

Remain spurred and keep fixed on your objectives, and you can effectively oversee and, surprisingly, switch type 1 diabetes.

Chapter 23: Conclusion And Final Thoughts On Reversing Type 1 Diabetes

The Power Of Mind And Body When Reversing Type 1 Diabetes:

The power of the mind and body can expect a section in managing the condition and dealing with by and large prosperity.

Coming up next are several different ways that the mind and body can help:

- Stress The chiefs: Tireless strain can antagonistically influence glucose levels, making it all the more difficult to administer Type 1 diabetes.

  Practicing pressure lessening methodologies like reflection, yoga, or significant breathing can help with controlling glucose levels.

- Work out: Standard dynamic work can help with additional creating insulin mindfulness, which consequently can help with overseeing glucose levels.

  Aim high 30 minutes of moderate action most days of the week.

- Shrewd counting calories: Eating a sensible eating schedule that is low in taking care of food sources, high in fiber, and consolidates a great deal of regular items, vegetables, and lean protein can help with controlling glucose levels and work on for the most part prosperity.

- Rest: Getting adequate rest is huge for all things considered, and it can similarly help with controlling glucose levels.

  Go all in significant stretches of rest each night.

It's basic to observe that while the mind and body can expect a section in directing Sort 1 diabetes, they should not be relied on as the sole strategy for treatment.

Individuals with Type 1 diabetes should work personally with their clinical benefits gathering to make a careful treatment plan that consolidates customary seeing of glucose levels, insulin treatment, and various medications relying upon the circumstance.

Taking Control Of Your Health When Reversing Type 1 Diabetes:

With legitimate administration and treatment, individuals with type 1 diabetes can have solid existences and keep up with great glucose control.

The following are a couple of steps you can take to deal with your sort 1 diabetes and work on your general wellbeing:

- Screen your glucose routinely: Monitoring your glucose levels consistently through self-checking can assist you with better comprehension how your body answers various food sources, active work, and different variables that can influence your glucose levels.

- Follow a solid eating regimen: Eating a reasonable eating routine that is high in fiber, low in added sugars and soaked fats, and plentiful in nutrients and minerals can assist you with keeping up with great glucose control and forestall difficulties related with type 1 diabetes.

- Work-out routinely: Active work can assist you with further developing your insulin responsiveness and control your glucose levels.

Intend to get somewhere around 30 minutes of moderate-power practice on most days of the week.

- Accept your insulin as endorsed: It's critical to adhere to your primary care physician's directions for taking insulin and to take it at the suggested times.

  In the event that you're experiencing difficulty dealing with your insulin routine, converse with your primary care physician about changing your treatment plan.

- Oversee pressure: Stress can affect your glucose levels, so it means a lot to track down solid ways of overseeing pressure, like through exercise, care, or other pressure the executives strategies.

- Get normal check-ups: Standard check-ups with your medical care group can assist you with observing your glucose control, check for inconveniences, and change your therapy plan on a case by case basis.

- Remain informed: Remain informed about the most recent improvements in type 1 diabetes exploration and medicines, and converse with your PCP about any new advances that might be applicable to your wellbeing.

Keep in mind, type 1 diabetes is a complicated and testing condition, yet with legitimate administration and a guarantee to great wellbeing, you can carry on with a full and dynamic life.

The Future Of Reversing Type 1 Diabetes:

Type 1 diabetes is a determined resistant framework disease that impacts a colossal number of people all over the planet.

While there is at present no answer for the condition, there are a couple of promising streets for research that could provoke better medications and, shockingly, a reasonable fix from here on out.

- Beta cell replacement treatment: This approach incorporates migrating pragmatic beta cells (the phones responsible for conveying insulin) into the body of a person with type 1 diabetes.

  While this treatment has shown promising results in clinical primers, it is still in its starting stages and isn't yet extensively open.

- Fundamental microorganism research: Researchers are examining the usage of undifferentiated creatures to make pragmatic beta cells that could be migrated into people with type 1 diabetes.

  This might perhaps give a sensible and long stretch solution for the disease.

- Fake Pancreas Structures: These systems mean to motorize the insulin transport process by using a blend of steady glucose checking (CGM) and an insulin siphon.

  They are planned to help people with type 1 diabetes stay aware of more unsurprising blood glucose levels, decline the rate of hypoglycemia, and work on commonly private fulfillment.

- Safe change: Experts are in like manner researching approaches to controlling the protected system to hold it back from pursuing and obliterating the beta cells in people with type 1 diabetes.

  This approach has shown promising results in animal examinations, and human primers are advancing.

- Quality treatment: This approach incorporates using quality treatment to override or fix the characteristics at risk for causing type 1 diabetes.

  This is still before all else periods of assessment, yet holds uncommon potential for what the future holds.

With everything taken into account, while there is still a great deal of work to be done, the fate of exchanging type 1 diabetes is looking more splendid as experts continue to make progress in developing new medications and medicines.

Regardless, it is fundamental to remember that these drugs are still in the first place periods of progression and may not be open for unfathomable use for a significant time span.